# A *Guide to*
# Biological Medicine

# A *Guide to* Biological Medicine

*A new approach to health and well-being
that combines noninvasive medical technology
with the body's natural healing power*

BIOLOGICAL MEDICINE
NETWORK
*Marion Foundation, Inc
Marion, Massachusetts.*
2002

Although the author and publisher have exhaustively researched all sources to ensure the accuracy and completeness of the information contained in this book, we assume no responsibility for errors, inaccuracies, omissions or any inconsistency herein. Any inaccurate characterizations of people, places or organizations are unintentional.

The information and procedures contained in this book are based on the research and the professional experience of the work at Paracelsus Klinik. This book has been published for information and reference uses only. It is not intended in any respect as a substitute for a visit to a qualified physician or other licensed health care practitioner. Every individual is genetically different, and no method of treatment is useful for everyone. If you have a medical problem, please consult a qualified physician or health care provider for diagnosis and treatment under their supervision. The publishers and author are not responsible for any adverse effects or consequences resulting from the use of any suggestions, procedures, techniques, protocols, remedies or preparations discussed in this book.

*Biological Medicine Network*
Marion Foundation, Inc.
3 Barnabas Road
Marion, Massachusetts 02738

First paperback edition

Distributed in the United States by Marion Foundation, Inc.

ISBN: 1-931188-06-8

# CONTENTS

*Preface vii*
*Acknowledgments xi*
*Introduction xiii*

Chapter 1: OVERVIEW OF BIOLOGICAL MEDICINE     I

Chapter 2: THE PRACTICE OF BIOLOGICAL MEDICINE     15

Chapter 3: A CLOSER LOOK AT DIAGNOSTIC AND     21
    TREATMENT METHODS

Chapter 4: PATIENT PERSPECTIVES     31

Conclusion: IS BIOLOGICAL MEDICINE FOR ME?     39

*APPENDICES*

*Appendix A About the Marion Foundation:*
    *Changing Ourselves, Changing the World 41*
*Appendix B About the Paracelsus Klinik 45*

*Glossary 49*
*Resource List 51*

# PREFACE

## Nathaniel's Story

*In 1993, when our son Nathaniel was about to turn thirteen, he was diagnosed with leukemia. His rapidly deteriorating condition required three rounds of chemotherapy, followed by a bone-marrow transplant from his sister. Complications from the transplant reduced his lung capacity by 50 percent. Essentially, the cancer was in remission, but we were told that his lung capacity would not recover.*

*We began to search for alternative treatments to reverse Nathaniel's loss of function, and we read about the Paracelsus Klinik in Switzerland. We spoke with the clinic director, Dr. Thomas Rau, a pioneer of European biological medicine.*

*When Nathaniel was well enough to travel, we took him to the clinic. Five years after that initial visit, Nathaniel is a college senior leading a normal, active life, with 97 percent of his lung capacity.*

*We are confident that biological medicine, with its emphasis on non-invasive diagnostic and treatment methods and the natural healing power of the body, is the principal reason for the remission of Nathaniel's disease and his current well-being.*

*Margie Baldwin*
Marion, Massachusetts

## Biological medicine

Biological medicine (sometimes called European biological medicine because of its origins) is the world's most complete model of holistic medicine.

> HOLISTIC MEDICINE: an approach to medicine that assumes that the human being is a functioning system operating in a "state of wholeness." Holistic medicine views all aspects of an individual – physical, mental, emotional, and spiritual – as interrelated. Any imbalance or disharmony is thought to cause sickness. The goal of holistic medicine is to correct the imbalance and restore "wholeness."

The basic approach to biological medicine is expressed in its name: *bio* (life) and *logical* (relating to knowledge). The foundation of biological medicine is the body's own "knowledge of life" — the body's innate wisdom regarding natural life forces within and around the individual.

In biological medicine, the practitioner and the individual work together to free the body's own natural healing systems. Also, because every person is unique, biological medicine treats the *individual*, not merely the disease and its symptoms.

When you are not feeling well or show symptoms of disease, you quite naturally want to feel as comfortable and confident as possible with your choice of physician and method of treatment. With this in mind, this book will help you explore biological medicine as an alternative approach to personal health and long-term well-being.

## Alternative medicine

Biological medicine is a form of alternative medicine. An increasing volume of information about alternative methods is entering mainstream American culture. For example, the two-volume *Health and Wellness Library* by Time-Life Books devotes nearly two hundred pages to alternative medicine, and the American Medical Association (AMA) is encouraging member physicians to become better informed regarding alternative medicine and to participate in appropriate studies.*

Still, many people are not getting the facts they need in order to make some very important decisions about their own health care. This lack of knowledge, plus anxiety associated with entering new and unfamiliar territory, often creates a reluctance to explore biological medicine (and other alternative health care methods). This is why it is important to answer some basic questions about biological medicine, which this guide does.

Biological medicine may not provide solutions for everyone's health care problems, but its essential philosophies and principles are sound and proven by the experiences of countless patients and practitioners, some of whom share their stories in these pages.

Ultimately, only you can determine if biological medicine makes sense for you, now or in the future. We simply hope that the information presented here will help you make better-informed decisions about your own health care and the health care needs of your loved ones.

## About this book

This book is designed for individuals who are considering biological medicine as a health care option or who are interested in increasing their knowledge of health care alternatives. Its four chapters are designed to provide useful information about biological medicine:

- Chapter 1: "Overview of Biological Medicine" explains the concepts behind biological medicine and compares it with conventional medicine.

---

* AMA Resolution #514, "Alternative (Complementary) Medicine," Reference Committee E, pp. 10–11.

- Chapter 2: "The Practice of Biological Medicine" provides information about the professionals who observe and practice the principles of biological medicine.
- Chapter 3: "A Closer Look at Diagnostic and Treatment Methods" discusses the methods practitioners use to diagnose and treat sickness.
- Chapter 4: "Patient Perspectives" profiles four individuals who share their personal experiences regarding the benefits of biological medicine.

The book concludes with a summary of factors to consider before you try biological medicine.

See the glossary for key terms and the appendices for profiles of the Biological Medicine Network at the Marion Foundation and the Paracelsus Klinik, and a list of resources you may wish to consult as you continue your journey.

# ACKNOWLEDGMENTS

The Marion Foundation would like to acknowledge the following individuals:

*Dede Cummings* for designing the book.

*Jay Frost,* a veteran medical writer, for preparing the manuscript, completing interviews, and editing the comments of others.

*Mike Henkle* for managing the project.

*Dr. Thomas Rau,* the leader of European biological medicine, for helping to enhance the lives of so many patients and making all of this possible.

We especially acknowledge all of those who contributed financially to help bring this document to publication:

*Michael and Margie Baldwin*
*David and Laurie Barrett*
*Chrissie and Charlie Bascom*
*Joan Brady*
*Johnnie and Buff Chace*
*Tim Cowles*
*Milo Fay*

*Peter and Lorraine Lieberson*
*M. Whitney and Phillip Long*
*John and Bonnie Lundberg*
*William and Elizabeth Oates*
*Phyllis Sondes*
*John and Gerry Tuten*

# INTRODUCTION

**Welcome to the world of biological medicine!**

Chances are, you are already familiar with the concepts of biological medicine, although you may not have heard the term. You may even have received health care that is consistent with the principles of biological medicine.

This is because biological medicine features some very *traditional* forms of health care (e.g., homeopathy, naturopathy, Chinese traditional medicine), combining these measures with aspects of contemporary medical practice and technology. The result is a truly integrated form of modern medicine that is well suited for everyone, regardless of age and health care history.

As you read this primer, you will learn that biological medicine:

- enhances quality of life
- produces desirable outcomes in a broad range of acute and chronic illnesses
- is useful for both healing and preventive health care
- can be cost-effective by producing desirable long-term outcomes and keeping patients out of doctors' offices, hospitals, and surgery wards
- is safe for adults and children

- is generally noninvasive (i.e., minimizes the medical need for invasive procedures such as surgery or radiation therapy)
- addresses long-term psychological and behavioral disorders (e.g., anxiety, depression, substance abuse, attention deficit disorder in children and adults)

Essentially, biological medicine integrates the following concepts into medical practice:

- All functions in a human being are dynamic, and all organs have the capability to rebuild themselves (at least to some extent) during a lifetime.
- We are all part of nature and intensely connected to nature, mainly through nutrition, which determines our "inner milieu."
- Biological medicine never treats diagnoses, but rather individuals; it rarely targets organs, but rather all of the body's functional systems.
- Biological medicine requires new ways of thinking about one's health — a belief that all disease has a purpose and that symptoms are never "diseases" per se, but rather signs that the body's regulation is out of sync. (This relates to the fact that we are all part of nature and respond in a natural manner to internal and external events.)

Perhaps most important for many patients, biological medicine is *safe*. It features comprehensive detoxification and stimulation techniques that rarely, if ever, cause side effects or peripheral damage to the body (such as might occur with chemotherapy or other aggressive treatments in conventional medicine).

Keep in mind that biological medicine can be effectively combined with conventional Western (or "allopathic") medical practices, often enhancing outcomes. This has been dramatically demonstrated in patients with cardiovascular disease, chronic inflammatory diseases (such as rheumatoid arthritis), and even severe cancers.

As you will learn, biological medicine is logical, is easy to understand, and treats patients as individuals. However, learning about biological medicine — and applying its principles in one's own life — involves change. Change begins with knowledge, and this primer is an excellent starting point to develop that knowledge.

*Dr. Thomas M. Rau*
Chief Medical Director
Paracelsus Klinik
Switzerland

# Chapter 1
# OVERVIEW OF
# BIOLOGICAL MEDICINE

## What is biological medicine?

As suggested in the preface, biological medicine utilizes a holistic approach to health and wellness that allows the human body to maximize its own innate healing powers.

A good way to understand biological medicine is to consider the methods conventional — or *allopathic* — physicians use to diagnose and treat disease, then compare those methods with the practice of biological medicine.

In general, conventional physicians are trained to identify symptoms of disease and to recommend treatments that eliminate or alleviate those symptoms. This approach often makes the patient feel better, but may not "cure" the disease or address the underlying condition(s) that allow the disease to manifest in the first place.

ALLOPATHIC: a system of therapeutics in which diseases are treated by producing a condition that is incompatible with or antagonistic to the disease and its symptoms. Examples of allopathic treatments include prescription pharmaceuticals, radiation, and surgery. All M.D.'s in the United States are licensed to practice allopathic medicine.

## Does biological medicine go beyond treating symptoms?

Yes. In addition to treating particular symptoms, biological medicine looks for the root causes of those symptoms. These root causes may consist of several factors that, over time, can allow disease-causing toxins to build up in the body. These factors include:

- diet
- lifestyle
- family history
- stress
- aging
- environmental factors
- trauma
- exposure to bacteria or virus

Looked at another way, our health often relates to how we feel, live, work, play, love, relax, socialize, and so on. Physiologically and psychologically, we all have "up-building" (regenerative) and "downgrading" (degenerative) forces within us, all of which are dependent on the factors listed above.

Biological medicine assesses the body's entire combination of physical, mental, emotional, and spiritual factors — everything that makes us tick — and tries to identify which combination of these factors may cause the body to be out of balance.

## Does biological medicine address these imbalances?

Yes, exactly. Practitioners of biological medicine are trained to identify these imbalances and recommend treatments that allow *nature* to take over and promote a restoration of balance.

These treatments support the body's "up-building" forces, help reverse degenerative activity, and promote long-term healing. They are generally noninvasive (surgery and radiation are examples of invasive treatments), and they rarely require the use of prescription drugs (which usually are not "natural" agents, often cause harmful side effects, and typically treat symptoms instead of the root causes of disease).

## Can you give an example of how conventional medicine and biological medicine might approach the same condition?

Let's take a simple example with which most of us are familiar: a child with an ear infection.

*Conventional medicine.* A conventional, allopathically trained pediatrician would normally perform the examination by checking the child's throat, listening to the lungs, and examining the ears. A typical examination might rule out flu, pneumonia, and other conditions. However, the doctor might notice swelling and redness in the child's ears and correctly diagnose an ear infection (*otitis media* in medical jargon).

In most cases, the pediatrician would prescribe an antibiotic, and perhaps recommend an analgesic or over-the-counter (OTC) cold medication to help relieve inflammation and pain. Chances are, in a day or two, the symptoms would disappear, and the child would resume normal activities.

Note that in this example the physician successfully alleviated symptoms (inflammation, pain). However, the physician also recommended the introduction of an antibiotic into the body. The drug killed the bacteria, exactly as it was supposed to do. The child, much to his or her satisfaction, experienced rapid relief from earache pain, but the antibiotic might also have destroyed millions of nonpathogenic bacteria essential for effective immune response.

Chances are, the drug actually interrupted the body's *natural* healing response. Thus, the child's immune system may not be any stronger the next time an infection occurs. This may increase the likelihood of future infections and create a dependency on antibiotics whenever the doctor suspects an infection.

*Biological medicine.* Now let's assume we have the same child with the same symptoms, except this time the parent takes the child to a biological medicine practitioner. Rather than zeroing in on symptoms, this practitioner would take a longer-term, bigger-picture assessment of the child's health.

This practitioner might use the same noninvasive diagnostic techniques to rule out serious disease, but he or she would probably spend a bit more time with the parent and child asking questions about home and school environment, the child's (and the family's) history of bacterial infections, the child's diet and historical use of antibiotics, and so on.*

The biological medicine practitioner would arrive at the same diagnosis: otitis media. However, instead of using the conventional "tried and true" method of prescrib-

NATUROPATHY: a system of medicine that treats health conditions by utilizing the body's inherent, natural ability to heal. Naturopathy aids the healing process by incorporating a variety of alternative methods based on the patient's individual needs. Diet, lifestyle, work, and personal history are all considered when determining a treatment regimen.

---

* It should be noted that some allopathic physicians will perform a comprehensive, detailed profile when diagnosing a patient. The point here is that virtually *all* biological medicine practitioners follow this procedure. Only in this manner can the practitioner recommend an appropriate treatment that goes beyond the rapid alleviation of symptoms.

ing an antibiotic and OTC medications, the practitioner would recommend less harmful treatments that would support and strengthen the body's natural healing power.

This practitioner would, of course, address the child's symptoms — no one wants to see a child suffer from pain. Accordingly, the practitioner might suggest a naturopathic ear oil (often available over-the-counter at retail drugstores and health food stores) to reduce pain as well as an herbal preparation, taken orally, to promote immune stimulation.

Symptomatic relief would probably occur quickly, but the complete, natural healing response might take longer. By allowing this natural healing response to occur, biological medicine allows the immune system to strengthen itself, perhaps increasing resistance to future infections.

## Is biological medicine effective for more serious, chronic diseases?

Yes. Biological medicine has an excellent track record for the successful treatment and management or elimination of serious, chronic, and potentially debilitating diseases. Asthma, allergies, diabetes, chronic fatigue syndrome, rheumatoid arthritis, depression, and even some cancers often respond to biological medicine.

Later in this book, you will learn more about how biological medicine addresses these serious diseases, sometimes in the words of patients.

## What are some other differences between biological medicine and conventional Western medicine?

Conventional medicine has historically attempted to manage the healing process by isolating, identifying, and measuring a broad

## Conventional medicine and biological medicine

| CONVENTIONAL MEDICINE | BIOLOGICAL MEDICINE |
|---|---|
| • Trains practitioners as specialists who tend to view the body as made up of separate systems (cardiovascular, endocrine, nervous, etc.) | • Trains practitioners to diagnose and treat holistically, i.e., to view the human being as a whole (physically, mentally, emotionally, spiritually) and each person as an individual. |
| • Generally diagnoses specific diseases (e.g., a general practitioner for flu or pneumonia, a cardiologist for heart disease, a psychiatrist for mental health, etc.) and treats symptoms (e.g., antibiotics for infections). | • Treats the body, mind, and spirit as an integral, interrelated system. Attempts to diagnose and treat the underlying cause(s) of disease within the context of the patient's life, family, work, relationships, lifestyle, etc. |
| • Tries to cure disease from the "outside in," e.g., by introducing pharmaceuticals to the body or performing invasive procedures. | • Attempts to promote true healing from the "inside out," e.g., by promoting and supporting the body's natural healing methods. |
| • Often utilizes "standardized" methods of care (usually based on results of clinical and empirical trials and clinical practice guidelines). | • Generally develops highly individualized treatment regimens (based on a holistic diagnosis that assesses genetic factors, environment, lifestyle, etc.) |
| • Focuses on prompt relief of symptoms and accelerated cures. | • Focuses on prompt relief of symptoms and rapid cures when appropriate, but takes a longer-term, holistic approach with an eye toward genuine and permanent healing. |

range of physiological, physical, and chemical reactions that can be documented by modern science. Usually, these measurements are assessed in clinical trials, such as those that compare and contrast the effects of new pharmaceutical agents on selected patient populations.

Conventional medicine also tends to isolate the various systems of the body, sometimes focusing on one system while de-emphasizing others. These systems include the cardiovascular, nervous, endocrine, pulmonary, gastrointestinal, musculoskeletal, and reproductive systems. This is one reason why conventional medicine has so many specialist physicians — cardiologists, rheumatologists, urologists, gynecologists, endocrinologists, and so on. Critics often refer to this approach as the "reductionist" model of Western medicine.

Biological medicine does not isolate or reduce the body into a series of discrete systems. Instead, it considers the human being as a comprehensive, integrated entity — body (and all its physiological systems, considered together), mind, spirit, and soul — and takes into account both the internal and external environments of the individual.

Biological medicine is capable of diagnosing diseases and conditions in a very precise manner because its practitioners take the time to map the connections between every system and organ in the body.

## Do practitioners of biological medicine utilize high-tech procedures?

When appropriate, yes.

Conventional medicine places a great deal of emphasis on techniques and technology. Because biological medicine focuses on the inherent, natural healing power of the body, you might think that it does not utilize modern technology. This is not true.

THERMOGRAPHY: a diagnostic technique that utilizes a thermalized (temperature-sensitive) wand, or thermister, to record skin temperature at 181 points on the body, first at standard room temperature, then at a lower temperature. Responses suggest organs and systems that are abnormally active and those that are depleted or not functioning properly.

In fact, many practitioners of biological medicine routinely use highly advanced noninvasive diagnostic procedures to help assess the overall performance of the body's interrelated systems. For example, a practitioner might order *computerized thermography* to evaluate the status of a patient's immune, digestive, cardiovascular, and autonomic nervous systems.

A practitioner might also take advantage of *darkfield microscopy* to assess cellular activity in the blood. This procedure magnifies live blood cells for detailed study of cell structure and function.

Biological medicine also utilizes technology in many other ways, including dried blood tests; heart-rate variability tests; and saliva, blood, and urine analysis.

## Is biological medicine considered a form of "alternative medicine"?

Yes. There is no one- or two-sentence definition of alternative medicine that satisfies everyone, but, in the United States, biological medicine is definitely considered a form of alternative medicine.

"While the term alternative medicine may conjure up some pretty exotic images, many of these therapies are more familiar than you think. If you've ever massaged your temples to ease a headache, applied an ice pack to a sprained ankle, or listened to your car radio to de-stress during a traffic jam, you've already practiced some simple natural healing techniques." — Bill Gottlieb, *New Choices in Natural Healing,* Rodale Press, 1995, p. 4.

In fact, biological medicine is made up of a rich array of techniques, modalities, and medical systems that may be unfamiliar to the majority of the public and are not practiced by most "mainstream" M.D.s. Consequently, these procedures are generally considered "alternatives" to those that Americans typically experience in the delivery of health care.

## What are some examples of alternative medicine?

There are many examples. Most (but not all) come to us from other parts of the world or from ancient healing traditions — settings in which they are/were not considered "alternative" at all.

For example, the use of herbs as medicine is a centuries-old practice found all over the world. In recent decades, herbal medicines have acquired a strong presence in the United States, where they can be purchased at pharmacies and health and nutrition centers and, in some cases, prepared at home.

Two examples of alternative medicine (holistic medicine and naturopathy) were introduced earlier. Other examples of alternative therapies include:

- **Acupressure.** Acupressure is a traditional Chinese therapeutic technique in which, using fingers or hands, pressure is applied to specific points on the body to alter the body's internal flow of life energy (referred to as "chi"), strengthening it, calming it, reducing it, increasing it, or eliminating blockages.
- **Acupuncture.** This is another traditional Chinese technique. With acupuncture, the flow of chi is released by the insertion of hair-thin needles at specific points on the body. Both acupuncture and acupressure are based on the traditional Chinese theory of meridians (see box).

- **Ayurvedic medicine.** Ayurvedic* theory suggests that diseases of the body are caused by stresses in the awareness, or consciousness, of the individual. These stresses lead to unhealthy practices, producing ill health. Treatments in ayurvedic medicine, which originated in India more than 5,000 years ago, include yoga-related body postures, breathing exercises, meditative techniques, special diets, and herbal remedies.

MERIDIANS: According to traditional Chinese medicine, acupressure and acupuncture points are aligned along fourteen energetic pathways within the body. These pathways are often called meridians.

Twelve of the meridians are bilateral (identical pathways on both sides of the body), and the other two are unilateral (running along the midline of the body).

Meridians do not correspond in any known way to the various anatomical and physiological principles taught in Western medical schools.

Practitioners of biological medicine often incorporate the meridian theory into their methods. For example, it is not unusual for a practitioner to successfully treat an intestinal dysfunction by repairing or removing a tooth that lies in the same meridian as the large intestine.

- **Homeopathy.** Homeopathy is a therapeutic system in which diseases are treated by substances that can cause symptoms of disease in a healthy person but that, when administered in minute doses, can cure those same symptoms. Most homeopaths practice constitutional homeopathy, a holistic approach that assumes that each person's "constitution" (physical, emotional, and mental factors) should be addressed in order to heal the disease.

- **Osteopathy.** Osteopathy focuses on addressing problems in the musculoskeletal system to correct and improve the general functioning of the body. A doctor of osteopathy (D.O.) combines manipulation of the joints, physical therapy, and recommendations for correcting posture. As a holistic form of health

---

* Interestingly, the term *ayurveda* derives from the Indian words meaning "life" and "knowledge." You'll recall that "biological" comes from the same root words (derived from Latin).

care, osteopathy also addresses emotional and psychological factors, nutrition, and lifestyle when addressing sickness and promoting good health.

- **Traditional Chinese medicine.** Traditional Chinese medicine is an ancient system of holistic health care that uses a variety of treatments including acupressure, acupuncture, herbal therapies, and massage, along with health-sustaining energetic body movement such as tai chi. Like biological medicine and many other alternative health care methods, Chinese medicine takes a holistic approach to health care by treating the entire body rather than individual systems.

Biological medicine synthesizes components of these (and sometimes other) forms of alternative medicine and combines these methods with modern, high-tech, noninvasive procedures.

## Does biological medicine apply to dental health, too?

Yes. While allopathic medicine generally views teeth as separate from the rest of the body and unrelated to overall health, dental treatment is often an essential element of biological medicine.

Root canals, implants, and dental amalgams (fillings) may contain heavy metals that can affect brain cells and the nervous system. Many of us have dental amalgams composed of toxic substances like mercury (which is so toxic that dentists must dispose of it as a hazardous waste) and palladium. In biological medicine, the removal of these amalgams from the mouth helps free the body of these toxins and is a fundamental part of the healing process.

Using a Panorex (a high-tech procedure that provides a detailed, panoramic picture of the teeth and entire jaw), biological medicine practitioners can obtain crucial information about the overall state of a person's health.

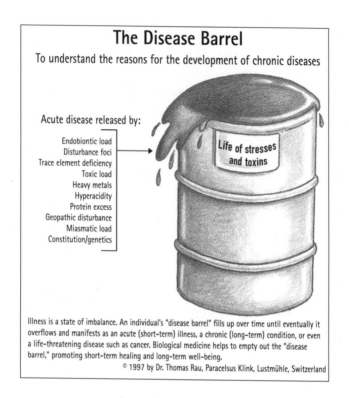

**The Disease Barrel**

To understand the reasons for the development of chronic diseases

Acute disease released by:

Endobiontic load
Disturbance foci
Trace element deficiency
Toxic load
Heavy metals
Hyperacidity
Protein excess
Geopathic disturbance
Miasmatic load
Constitution/genetics

Life of stresses and toxins

Illness is a state of imbalance. An individual's "disease barrel" fills up over time until eventually it overflows and manifests as an acute (short-term) illness, a chronic (long-term) condition, or even a life-threatening disease such as cancer. Biological medicine helps to empty out the "disease barrel," promoting short-term healing and long-term well-being.

© 1997 by Dr. Thomas Rau, Paracelsus Klink, Lustmühle, Switzerland

## How important is the removal of toxins in biological medicine?

Very important. This becomes easier to understand when you consider the body as a "disease barrel." This analogy, developed by Dr. Thomas Rau, a pioneer of biological medicine, compares the human body's susceptibility to disease with an ordinary waste barrel. This is our "disease barrel."

Our body has the ability to accept and respond to an enormous variety of stresses and toxins. However, if allowed to accumulate, these factors can exceed the body's ability to handle them. When this happens, the body's natural balancing system (called "homeostasis") becomes compromised.

Put simply, illness is a state of imbalance. As Dr. Rau states, an individual's disease barrel fills up over time until eventually it overflows and manifests as an acute (short-term) illness, a chronic (long-term) condition, or even a life-threatening disease such as cancer. Biological medicine helps to empty out the disease barrel, promoting short-term healing and long-term well-being.

## What specific acute and chronic illnesses can be treated with biological medicine?

The holistic biological medicine model is suitable for the treatment of many acute and virtually all chronic diseases, including:

- allergies (including hidden food or environmental allergies)
- asthma
- cancer and tumor diseases
- cardiovascular disease (including angina pectoris and hypertension)
- chronic fatigue syndrome
- fungal infections (e.g., candidiasis)
- hay fever
- immunosuppressive disorders
- intoxication and amalgam problems
- neuralgias
- neurodermatitis
- rheumatoid arthritis
- allergic rhinitis
- stomach and colon disorders (e.g., colitis, constipation, Crohn's disease, diarrhea, digestive problems, flatulence, ulcers)
- tooth and jaw infections

IS BIOLOGICAL MEDICINE SAFE? Yes. In fact, most biological medicine practitioners and their patients consider biological medicine to be safer than conventional medicine. This is because biological medicine generally avoids the use of invasive procedures (such as surgery) and the use of mainstream prescription pharmaceuticals (which may introduce chemicals and toxins that do not naturally occur in the body and cause uncomfortable side effects).

In cases where surgery is required, pre- and post-operative procedures may be performed using biological medicine principles. For example, practitioners of biological medicine do not recommend the use of metal staples (which may introduce toxic substances into the body and restrict energy flow) to close incisions.

When the crisis of disease occurs, conventional medical procedures often zero in to eradicate symptoms, not to eliminate the causes. While this approach has an important place — and is indeed essential — in the menu of health care options, biological medicine strongly asserts that unless the causes are addressed, crises will recur, as we see in chronic diseases such as asthma, cardiovascular disease, rheumatoid arthritis, and even cancer.

## Is biological medicine appropriate for children?

Acute and chronic disease and behavioral disorders of children can be treated effectively and gently by biological medicine. Children are very often highly responsive to the natural approaches of biological medicine.

## How can I be confident that biological medicine works?

No system of medicine can guarantee success for every condition in every patient. What works for one person may be less effective for another. Each system — conventional or alternative — is well suited to address certain health care conditions.

In biological medicine, an individual's willingness to take responsibility for his or her own healing is part of the process. Consequently, it is important to be well-informed.

We hope that the principles outlined in this guidebook will help you make appropriate choices for your particular situation.

## Chapter 2
# THE PRACTICE OF BIOLOGICAL MEDICINE

### Who practices biological medicine?

A variety of health care professionals practice biological medicine.

Keep in mind that biological medicine is not considered a medical specialty in the same sense that we think of family practice, cardiology, gastroenterology, urology, and other medical disciplines as specialties.

The fact is, virtually all types of practitioners can incorporate the principles of biological medicine into their practices. A variety of healthcare professionals, including conventional physicians, chiropractors, dentists, doctors of osteopathy and homeopathy, and nurse practitioners can use techniques of biological medicine when diagnosing and treating patients.

### Are these professionals licensed to practice biological medicine?

There is currently no special licensing requirement for the incorporation of biological medicine in medical practice.

Medical practitioners are licensed to practice in their individual disciplines by appropriate licensing boards and professional accreditation organizations. For example, a general practitioner must be licensed in general practice (or family medicine), and an obstetrician-gynecologist (ob-gyn) must be licensed by the appropriate ob-gyn licensing board. In the United States, most medical licensing is performed at the state level — each of the fifty states has its own licensing boards.

If you have any concerns about the qualifications of any medical practitioner, you should investigate his or her background and be aware of any licensing requirements in your state or county. Ask for detailed information about diagnostic methods, treatments, and procedures the practitioner uses, and remember that you are in charge of decisions about your own health care.

## Are practitioners of biological medicine required to have any special kind of formal training in biological medicine?

Medical professionals can incorporate whatever degree of biological medicine they feel comfortable with into their practices, and anyone who utilizes principles of biological medicine should have some formal training that meets their individual requirements and professional goals.

Formal training and certification in biological medicine is currently available at the Paracelsus Klinik in Switzerland. Periodically, training programs are offered in the United States at the Paracelsus Foxhollow Clinic in Kentucky and the Marion Foundation in Massachusetts.

## Are practitioners of biological medicine graduates of medical school?

Some are. All licensed physicians (M.D.s) who treat patients in the United States are graduates of accredited medical schools, regardless of whether or not they utilize biological medicine methods.

Other medical professionals (i.e., nonphysicians, such as psychologists, chiropractors, physician assistants, and nurse practitioners) who use biological medicine techniques in their practices must possess accreditation credentials issued by the appropriate licensing boards in their specific disciplines.

TRAINING AND CERTIFICATION IN BIOLOGICAL MEDICINE: To further the understanding and practice of biological medicine, the Marion Foundation has held training seminars for practitioners and created the Biological Medicine Network (BMN). Many U.S. practitioners have completed the Marion Foundation's two-year certification program in biological medicine and are affiliated with the BMN.

## Where can I find a practitioner of biological medicine?

There are several hundred physicians and other practitioners in the United States who currently incorporate biological medicine principles into their practices.

If a health care provider gave you this publication, chances are that he or she uses biological medicine methods or knows someone who does.

For information about where to find a practitioner of biological medicine in your area, consult the resource list at the back of this book.

# Can I consult a practitioner of biological medicine and still continue to see my personal physician?

ONE PHYSICIAN'S OPINION: "In my work as a physician — and as a practitioner of alternative medicine — I am constantly reminded of the importance of keeping an open mind when it comes to finding out what's best for my patients. Years of experience have shown me that no single approach to health care has all the answers; the search for healing solutions often requires a willingness to look beyond one remedy or system of treatment.

"At the same time, I also feel a deep responsibility to be selective — to recognize important distinctions among the vast array of treatment options available. Because the same therapy can affect different patients in different ways, an approach that works for one patient may do nothing for another.

"My job, then, is not just to seek out which remedies are available or safe, but to prescribe the course of treatment that best suits the patient's condition and lifestyle. I've discovered, though, that I can't do this job alone. Whatever the therapy, patients respond dramatically better to treatment when they take an active, confident role in their own health care."*

— JEFFREY MIGDOW, M.D.

* Health and Wellness, The Southwestern Company, 2000, p. 8. © Time Life Inc.

Yes. If you are considering biological medicine as an alternative or complement to the care you currently receive, we recommend that you share your thoughts and health care goals with your personal physician. Tell your physician about the options you are considering.

A dedicated physician will support your efforts to learn more about biological medicine and other types of alternative health care (see box at left). In some cases, your personal physician may even refer you to a professional who is familiar with biological medicine.

For most individuals, biological medicine is not an either/or proposition. Biological medicine offers an alternative to conventional medicine, often in a complementary manner.

It is up to you to decide the extent to which you want to use biological medicine — to treat a specific disease or condition or to incorporate biological medicine into your life on a long-term basis.

## Are consultations and treatments in biological medicine covered by health insurance or managed care plans?

Possibly. It depends on the state you live in and your insurance plan. A few states and many health plans are expanding coverage to include some types of alternative health care.

For example, Blue Cross of Washington and Alaska offers a plan entitled "AlternaPath," which covers licensed naturopathic doctors. These physicians may employ principles of biological medicine in their services, which may be covered by Blue Cross, although a patient should always confirm this prior to a medical appointment.

In many situations, health plans require that treatment for alternative medicine be defined as "medically necessary." Usually, a conventional physician, who functions as a "gatekeeper," decides what particular treatment is medically necessary. Keep in mind that some physicians who determine medical necessity may be biased against some alternative medicine practices.

Recently, in response to consumer demand, as well as to evidence that alternative medicine works for many people, coverage for alternative health care options has become more common.

If you are considering biological medicine and are concerned about insurance coverage, ask your practitioner if he or she has experience with your particular insurer regarding reimbursement for alternative health care. If the answer is no, contact your health insurance representative and obtain current information about possible coverage for alternative medical treatments.

Be specific about any preventive measures, diagnostic procedures, and treatments that you are thinking about. If it turns out that your plan does not cover these items, it may be worth your time and money to shop around for a different insurance plan. You may find a plan that is better suited for your health care needs. If you are unsuccessful in your efforts to obtain coverage, you will be required to pay out-of-pocket for expenses associated with biological medicine.

## Can I go to the Paracelsus Klinik in Switzerland or the Paracelsus Foxhollow Clinic in Kentucky to receive care?

Yes. Right now, these two centers provide comprehensive diagnostic and treatment options for biological medicine. Their physicians, dentists, therapists, and other professionals provide a broader range of experience in biological medicine than at any other facility in the world. For more information about these two clinics, visit their websites:

- Paracelsus Klinik: www.paracelsus.ch/e/index.htm
- Paracelsus Foxhollow Clinic: www.foxhollow.com

## *Chapter 3*
# A Closer Look at Diagnostic and Treatment Methods

### How does a practitioner of biological medicine diagnose disease or other ailments?

As mentioned earlier, biological medicine takes a holistic view of the human body and does not isolate or reduce the body into separate systems. Thus, an assessment of the functioning of each of the body's systems is essential to diagnosis. Based upon this information, treatments are designed to help revitalize organs and systems so that the individual can *resist* disease and prevent recurrences.

### Isn't this the same thing that conventional and holistic practitioners do?

To an extent, yes, but biological medicine is different. Conventional medicine is designed to identify disease and treat symptoms. Rarely, however, do conventional physicians — and even practitioners of holistic medicine — attempt to detect subtle systemic imbalances that can predict major illness. Most practitioners of biological medicine take the time to do this.

## What diagnostic techniques does the practitioner use to identify these subtle imbalances?

The practitioner usually begins with a comprehensive interview, a physical examination, and selected medical tests.

Tests may include pulse reading; analyses of blood, urine, and saliva; dental and skin examinations; hearing and vision tests; cardiovascular tests; kinesthetic evaluation (see box); and others.

KINESTHETICS: Kinesthetics refers to the science of movement. In biological medicine, a practitioner often assesses the ways in which a patient perceives movement, weight, position, etc. The purpose is to identify changes in the angles of joints, which may be indicative of disease.

Together, the interview, exam, and tests enable the practitioner to customize a treatment program that matches your individual needs.

Generally, you can expect a biological medicine practitioner to conduct what is sometimes called a "biological terrain assessment" during diagnosis.

A terrain assessment evaluates the health status of an individual through analysis of the blood, urine, and saliva.

## What are some of the specific diagnostic measures used in the "terrain assessment"?

A terrain assessment evaluates the health status of an individual through analysis of the blood, urine, and saliva. Prior to the tests, a patient is asked to fast for twelve hours — avoiding even toothpaste and the use of cosmetics before the tests are administered.

Practitioners use the results of these tests to determine how well the body absorbs nutrients and produces energy. While these tests do not identify specific diseases, they can provide an excellent profile of overall health. Blood tests can help determine the presence of environmental toxins in the body. Analysis of saliva reveals information about liver function. Urinalysis reveals the level of kidney function and the ability of the kidneys to filter toxins from the body.

Other diagnostic measures might include computerized thermography and darkfield microscopy (both described in chapter 1).

## How does biological medicine attempt to restore health?

For the practitioner of biological medicine, helping to restore a patient's health is a threefold process:

1. The practitioner performs an appropriate combination of diagnostic tests to identify blockages, imbalances, and potential toxins.

2. The practitioner works with the patient to develop treatments that systematically remove stored toxins that may be obstructing energy flow and the balance among systems and organs.

3. The practitioner recommends treatments, dietary changes, lifestyle alterations, etc., that will help stimulate the responsiveness of all the body's systems or calm and balance overactive systems.

## Can you provide an example?

Here's an excellent example provided by a patient who suffered from chronic asthma.

A PATIENT'S STORY: I was incapacitated by my asthma for nearly six years. I slept twenty hours a day and took six different medications three times a day, all to no avail. Finally, I went to Paracelsus Foxhollow Clinic in Kentucky, under the care of Dr. Robert Zieve, a practitioner of biological medicine. Foxhollow currently operates the most comprehensive biological medicine clinic in the United States and treats many people from all over the country who suffer from chronic disease.

When you go to see a biological practitioner, you talk about *everything* that's affecting you. My doctor spent hours talking with me, not just minutes like other doctors. For me, Dr. Zieve ordered a computerized thermography to assess how well my immune, digestive, autonomic nervous, and circulatory systems were functioning. A technician measured about 100 points on my body, first at normal room temperature, then in a cooler room, to determine how my skin, nervous system, and corresponding organs were functioning. These responses reflected where my body's functions were impaired, and, in my case, my liver and adrenal functions registered as weak.

Next, Dr. Zieve looked at my blood through a darkfield microscope, a remarkable German invention that shows live blood cells against a dark background, which allows a close look at cell activity. He noticed that my white blood cells were sluggish, suggesting an impaired immune system.

The diagnosis? Food allergies.

Dr. Zieve advised me to eliminate wheat and dairy products from my diet and to apply castor oil packs to my liver — a naturopathic treatment — at home. He also prescribed naturopathic remedies to help detoxify my liver and revitalize my adrenal glands.

Over the next six months, I was able to reduce and finally eliminate my asthma medications. Today, I have enough energy to work full days in my restaurant business, baby-sit my grandchildren in the evening, and bake wheat-free breads and rolls for my on-line business.

*Dr. Zieve says he has observed this kind of healing many times in his practice.*

**The example above is for an asthma patient. What if I were diagnosed with another disease, say, diabetes or even cancer?**

The principles are the same, although the practitioner will develop specific diagnostic procedures and treatments that match the unique needs of each patient. Chapter 4 describes the experiences of patients with different diseases, including cancer.

**What if I have a relatively simple ailment, such as the common cold, a seasonal flu, or an upper respiratory infection? Is biological medicine appropriate?**

Biological medicine can help reduce the frequency of these events or help prevent them altogether. Biological medicine remedies can help alleviate the symptoms of many acute and chronic ailments.

Keep in mind, however, that certain common ailments, such as the common cold, represent a natural way to rid the body of harmful organisms and *strengthen the immune system*. In these cases, most biological medicine practitioners will take a longer-term view by addressing symptoms while allowing the body's natural healing process to take its own course.

**What treatment methods are used by practitioners of biological medicine?**

Let's take a closer look at some of the treatment methods commonly used in biological medicine:

## Homeopathy

Homeopathy (introduced in chapter 1) is an inexpensive, nontoxic system of medicine used by hundreds of millions of people worldwide. It is especially effective for treating chronic illnesses that fail to respond to conventional treatment. Homeopathic methods are well suited for self-care for conditions such as the common cold and flu.

TESTING HOMEOPATHIC REMEDIES: Most homeopathic remedies have been evaluated in medical trials in which healthy subjects receive undiluted or slightly diluted doses of substances known to cause sickness.

During the tests, clinicians assess the subjects' physical, mental, and emotional responses to determine the range of symptoms produced by the substance.

Responses have been recorded over many years and published in a reference document that provides homeopathic practitioners with evidence for their decision-making.

Homeopathy is a method of healing based on the idea that "like cures like." In other words, an agent that might cause certain symptoms of illness in a healthy person can cure the same symptoms in someone who is sick.

Homeopathic remedies are derived from plant, mineral, and animal extracts that are highly diluted using precise methods that eliminate toxicity while increasing a substance's potential to relieve symptoms or cure disease.

Homeopathic remedies are most effective in the treatment of ailments that have not yet caused severe damage to body organs and systems and for conditions that require the chronic use of conventional pharmaceuticals. Allergies and arthritis are two examples of these conditions.

In the United States, homeopathic remedies are acknowledged and regulated by the federal Food and Drug Administration. Many remedies are available over the counter at retail pharmacies, while some must be prescribed by a licensed practitioner.

## *Ayurvedic medicine*

The primary focus of ayurvedic medicine is preventive health care, although ayurvedic methods can provide relief for many chronic ailments. Medical researchers are currently studying the effects of ayurvedic treatments for arthritis, cancer, high cholesterol, Parkinson's disease, diabetes, and chemical addictions.

Ayurvedic practitioners use a variety of treatments and methods for healing, which are usually separated into two categories: constitutional and therapeutic. Constitutional treatments involve lifestyle changes, breathing exercises, and adjustments to sleeping and eating habits. A practitioner may also recommend dietary changes that include certain herbal supplements. Therapeutic treatments include natural medicinal remedies and cleansing procedures (such as therapeutic vomiting and herbal enemas).

## *Chiropractic*

Like other aspects of biological medicine, chiropractic care assumes that the body has an innate self-healing ability and always seeks homeostasis. Chiropractic theory holds that the central nervous system plays a key role in maintaining homeostasis, but that certain misalignments of the joints or irregularities of motion can interfere with nervous system activity, causing pain and possible deterioration of general health. By manipulating muscles and joints — especially the spine — chiropractors readjust these irregularities, enhancing neuromuscular function and restoring homeostasis.

Until recently, chiropractic was considered a form of alternative medicine. In recent years, chiropractic has gained wide acceptance in the United States Chiropractic services are now covered by Medicare and most major insurance and managed care plans.

Chiropractic care is considered beneficial in the treatment of arthritis, asthma, back pain, repetitive motion disorders (e.g., carpal tunnel syndrome), chronic fatigue syndrome, headache, tendonitis, and many other common ailments.

### Neural therapy

Neural therapy involves the injection of homeopathic remedies into the body's acupuncture points. The remedies are introduced into the body's autonomic nervous system, which regulates all involuntary bodily functions (such as heartbeat and respiration). The autonomic nervous system features sensors throughout the skin, and thus provides pathways for the delivery of medicine to the body's key organs and systems.

In biological medicine, practitioners use a mild anesthetic (e.g., lidocaine or procaine) as the basic ingredient in an injection, adding one or more homeopathic or other natural remedies, selected by the practitioner, according to the diagnosis.

The injection points are carefully identified according to sources of blockage or disturbance diagnosed by the practitioner. For example, injecting lung points can help address asthma or lung disorders, while injecting certain bladder or kidney points can help enhance adrenal output and improve kidney function.

## What role does dentistry play in biological medicine?

Conventional medicine has arbitrarily separated dentistry from medicine — an unusual distinction, since the mouth and teeth are essential parts of the body. Consequently, conventional physicians rarely consider the mouth and teeth when attempting to diagnose a problem.

On the other hand, practitioners of biological medicine emphasize that the mouth and teeth can have a profound impact on what occurs in other parts of the body. Because of the meridian system, each tooth connects to a specific organ or system in the body. Accordingly, an unhealthy tooth on the heart meridian could, along with other factors (such as age or poor diet), contribute to heart disease.

Consider root canals, which are widely used in modern dentistry. A completed root canal may harbor a hidden infection that can undermine the immune system by forcing it to fight a chronic, low-grade infection. The same root canal may also weaken corresponding meridian organs. Conversely, weakened organs can affect the health of a corresponding tooth, sometimes causing decay.

Consider, too, the presence of mercury, widely used in amalgam fillings. Mercury is a known poison that in many circumstances must be disposed of according to stringent requirements. Small amounts of mercury may leak from fillings and circulate throughout the body, where toxicity can cause chronic fatigue, depression, and joint pain.

Biological medicine can identify mercury toxicity through a variety of tests. Mercury can then be removed, according to strict guidelines by a dentist trained in the procedure. In addition, biological practitioners often recommend oral supplements that can help remove mercury from the organs and systems of the body.

Both the Paracelsus Klinik and the Paracelsus Foxhollow Clinic feature dentists on staff whose services in the diagnosis and treatment of disease complement those of physicians.

## What can I do on my own to promote the healing process?

To optimize the value of your biological medicine treatment, it is important to follow dietary guidelines, take appropriate supplements, follow an exercise or bodywork routine (see box), and perform other activities recommended by your practitioner.

Because biological medicine assumes the integration of mind and body, identifying and addressing core emotional issues are also essential for successful treatment. Biological medicine can call upon a wide range of healing therapies that target the emotions, including homeopathy, imagery, meditation, and psychotherapy.

BODYWORK: Bodywork refers to a variety of techniques that promote relaxation and treat certain ailments, especially musculoskeletal disorders. Treatment techniques usually involve some combination of massage, movement awareness, structural realignment, and energy balancing. Most bodywork regimens take a holistic approach to care and include treatment of both mind and body.

Gaining familiarity with the underlying theories supporting biological medicine will help enhance your understanding of how and why its diagnostic and treatment techniques work. You may also find it useful to learn about the experiences related by patients of biological medicine, such as the patients profiled in the next chapter.

## *Chapter 4*
# PATIENT PERSPECTIVES

ONE OF THE BEST WAYS to assess the value of a particular approach to medicine is to hear the first-person stories of patients. Here, in their own words, are the experiences of four individuals whose lives have been changed by biological medicine.

### Elizabeth McBride, *68, retired university advisor, Albuquerque, N.M. (breast cancer)*

I was diagnosed with stage II breast cancer that had metastasized in both sides. My surgeon recommended a lumpectomy, followed by chemotherapy and radiation to eradicate the cancer. But I was horrified by my poor chances — just 10 to 20 percent chance for improvement with 40 to 60 percent chance of recurrence. Plus, the treatments would basically destroy my body's systems while trying to kill the cancer.

Fortunately, a friend of mine who is an advocate of biological medicine provided me with some articles. I made the decision to choose biological medicine, over the strong opposition of my family members — including my son, who is a doctor, and his wife, who is a breast cancer surgeon. My experience suggests that, because biological medicine is not considered conventional, you should be prepared for opposition.

I scheduled a stay at the Paracelsus Klinik in Switzerland, but there was a two-month wait. In the meantime, I consulted with Dr. Fitzpatrick, a naturopathic physician in Santa Fe who is familiar with Dr. Rau. I also viewed videotaped presentations of Dr. Rau in which he stressed detoxification of the body's systems and rebuilding of the immune system in a nonharmful, noninvasive manner—exactly the opposite of chemotherapy and radiation. I saw biological medicine as a positive approach toward the problem, not a negative one.

I was still a little uncertain and had time to back out, but ultimately I flew to Switzerland for the first of four visits. You'll meet a lot of other patients who are all very, very nice people.

My first reaction was amazement at the extremely modern, high-tech equipment at the clinic. Next, I was surprised by the extent of testing they do — far more than in conventional medicine — to get an individualized profile of a patient.

Tests included blood tests, circular x-rays, darkfield microscopy, computerized thermography, and others, including a detailed dental examination. I have nice teeth, but examination of the roots and analysis of the various meridians revealed some problems along the meridian that went from certain teeth to the stomach via the breasts.

Another thing they noticed was that my mercury levels were off the charts, so I had amalgam fillings removed, as well as five teeth from the back of my mouth. This was all done seamlessly using "space-age" dentistry techniques and was done with the understanding that heavy metal poisoning is a key factor in the development of cancer.

Dr. Rau then performed neural therapy, which required a series of injections into the breasts, neck, and thyroid gland. There were many other treatments as well. One was hyperthermia, which raises the body's temperature for four hours, creating an environment in which cancer cells cannot survive. I felt totally safe, as I was monitored by a nurse during the session.

I was also asked if I was doing my "inner work." This is a big part of biological medicine, but it is not forced on you. Many cancer patients have issues related to religion, spirituality, and psychology. There is a psychiatrist on staff to help you address any mental health issues.

My initial session at Paracelsus was for three weeks, and subsequent visits have been for two weeks. When I returned after my first visit, my cancer was in complete remission, but I chose to return every six months to be monitored. I am happy to say it is still in remission, and I am living an active, normal life.

I continue post-treatments here at home with Dr. Fitzpatrick, who provides me with naturopathic infusions and injections, along with vials of homeopathic remedies that I take every day. My diet is restricted — no animal protein, no dairy products, all organic vegetables. It is worth all of this to stay active and healthy.

When I am asked about the cost of biological medicine, I say, yes, it was somewhat expensive, but the dental treatments in Europe were far less expensive than what you would pay here. And the overall cost of treatment was far less than the cost of chemotherapy and radiation alone. Of course, insurance in the United States would have covered these services, but at what price to my overall health and survival?

If you don't think you can afford it, you have to ask yourself, what's your life worth? As a retiree from a university job, I am not wealthy, but for me my experience was well worth it.

**Serita Winthrop, *58, social worker, New York City (eczema)***

I was diagnosed with eczema* when I was just three months old. As I got older, I learned that my condition was chronic, a lifelong condition that flared up periodically, always when I was under a lot of stress. I had three month long hospital stays at ages three, ten, and twenty-three. That last one was three months after my first marriage, and it was at that time that I was given injections and pills of cortisone as well as creams.

It wasn't until I was fifty that I discovered I had severe osteoporosis as a result of the cortisone. When I had a severe outbreak after my second marriage, I wanted to avoid cortisone but was desperate and enormously relieved when Dr. Rau at the Paracelsus Klinik told me that removing the metal fillings from my teeth was very likely to help with the clearing of my eczema. He also treated the osteoporosis.

The combination of treatments that I had under care at the Paracelsus Klinik and the addressing of emotional and spiritual issues, brought my skin under control. I am learning to listen better to my feelings, though my skin remains a barometer. (I actually had to leave my second marriage in order for my skin to clear completely.) It took a couple of years for the metal to leave my system, but Dr. Rau had warned me that it would take that long.

I will always feel enormous gratitude to Dr. Rau whose intuitive powers are part of what make him a brilliant healer.

---

* An inflammatory skin condition characterized by redness, itching, oozing, crusting, and scaling.

### Richard Griscom, *66, semi-retired attorney, Galisteo, N.M.*
*(prostate cancer)*

I was undergoing a routine physical in October 1999. My PSA (prostate-specific antigen) test was normal, but my internist suspected that my prostate gland was too large and recommended a biopsy. He referred me to a specialist, and as a result of the biopsy, I was diagnosed with prostate cancer.

I consulted with various doctors and decided upon a course of therapy that included hormone treatments in November and radiation beginning in January 2000. However, before that happened, I talked with a physician who suggested that a visit to the Paracelsus Klinik might be more beneficial than radiation. So I scheduled a three-week visit to Paracelsus in March.

I completed a course of neural therapy, as well as magnetic therapy, which is a treatment of about twenty minutes during which magnetic fields surround the area of the cancer. Localized heat therapy was also part of my regimen, and I received ozone treatments as well. I had lots of dental work done, including removal of mercury fillings and three teeth. I made a follow-up visit to Paracelsus in early 2001.

I continue to consult with my personal physicians, with an oncologist who is neutral regarding a patient's choice of conventional versus alternative methods, and with a homeopathic physician here in New Mexico. I am on high intravenous doses of vitamin C, as well as other homeopathic medications that neutralize acidity and promote an environment in which the cancer cannot grow.

As a result of all this, I am healthy and active, and I never had to have the radiation.

### Arnold "Buff" Chace, 54, *businessman, Providence, R.I.* *(bladder cancer)*

In November 1998, I noticed blood in my urine and went to a urologist for a diagnosis. Under general anesthesia, I underwent an examination of the urethra, during which a tumor was discovered and excised for analysis. This proved to be the source of blood in the urine, and I was diagnosed with transitional cell carcinoma, a cancer for which, if it reappeared, the outlook was not good. The literature suggests that this type of cancer has a 75 percent chance of recurring.

When I asked how and why I might have contracted the cancer, the doctors asked if I worked in a tannery or smoked. When I answered no to both questions, they said they did not know. Their best advice was to repeat the diagnostic procedure every three months to check for recurrence, something that I still do today.

However, I was not satisfied and wanted to know what steps I could take to prevent recurrence. I was familiar with Margie Baldwin at the Marion Foundation and was aware of the situation with her son, Nathaniel.* I knew that after Nathaniel visited the Paracelsus Klinik and Dr. Thomas Rau, his condition improved significantly. So I did some research on Paracelsus and because of their interest in why things occur, I decided that this was my type of place.

I went to Paracelsus in January 1999 for a two-week stay. I was found to have heavy-metal toxicity, as well as an immune system that was compromised and very weak. Dr. Rau initiated a number of natural therapies and made many adjustments in the regimen to ensure that they were effective. I also had all of my mercury amalgam fillings removed and replaced.

With the help of Paracelsus, I adopted a different approach to diet — mostly vegetarian — that would promote "flushing" my system

* See "Nathaniel's story," in the Preface.

of all the heavy metals. Dr. Rau calls it "changing the milieu" to one that promotes better health.

There were also regular heat treatments, mistletoe injections, colon-cleansing procedures, ozone treatments, and neural therapy, including injections into the bladder. Observing the principles of the meridian system, Dr. Rau identified a splitting tooth that related to the bladder — the site of the cancer. The tooth was injected as a way of rejuvenating it.

I have taken various vitamins and minerals and make a point to exercise to produce a sweat, which helps rid the body of toxins.

It's interesting to note that mercury levels in my blood have actually increased, which just indicates how much mercury was in the tissue and needs to be expelled.

The bottom line is that since my first visit to Paracelsus more than three years ago, there has been no recurrence of the cancer. I am totally sold on this approach to health care, and I am particularly impressed by Dr. Rau's open approach and willingness to employ whatever works. He does not follow a strict approach to treatment, is not set in his ways at all, and is into results.

Because this holistic approach to medicine addresses the psychological component of disease as well, I have taken steps to change the ways in which I deal with stress.

I have been so impressed that I have referred several family members and friends to Paracelsus for everything from hyperthyroidism and an oversized wisdom tooth to breast cancer and other cancers. I really believe that this is a very beneficial approach to one's health.

## Conclusion
# IS BIOLOGICAL MEDICINE FOR ME?

WHEN YOU ASSUME THE ROLE of patient, you need to feel as comfortable and confident as possible with your choice of practitioner and methods of diagnosis and treatment. Consideration of appropriate health care choices is an intensely personal journey for everyone, from the selection of over-the-counter medications at a retail drugstore to decisions regarding treatment for debilitating and life-threatening diseases.

Biological medicine is perhaps not the answer for everybody, but its philosophies and principles are sound and provide worthwhile health care solutions for millions of people worldwide. The fact that you have read this guidebook suggests that you have taken the first step toward making a commitment to a deeper level of personal health care that can generate rewards for a lifetime — hopefully, a longer lifetime.

We hope the overview we have presented here will help you make informed decisions about your own health care, beginning right now.

Please utilize the resources in the appendix to find additional information about biological medicine and types of alternative health care, or contact the Biological Medicine Network at the Marion Foundation to learn more about the Paracelsus Klinik in Switzerland, the Paracelsus Foxhollow Clinic in Kentucky, or a biological medicine practitioner near you.

## Appendix A
# ABOUT THE MARION FOUNDATION:
### *Changing Ourselves, Changing the World*

THE MARION FOUNDATION is a nonprofit organization based in Marion, Massachusetts. The purpose of the organization is to broaden understanding of the universe in order to generate new choices for addressing global problems.

We believe that enriching ways of knowing ourselves and our world will expand possibilities for affecting change. Such new possibilities are greatly needed. We believe that being human is a far more mysterious and beautiful experience than Western culture has encouraged us to recognize.

The Marion Foundation is a "gathering foundation". It is not financially endowed. We gather ideas, people, and money to connect them in new, more transformative ways through:

*Ideas.* We search for and share ideas that change how we see, understand, experience, and act in the world.

*People.* We seek to deepen relationships with individuals and organizations as they become partners in our learning and actions.

*Money.* We seek to understand how humanity and society are affected by the idea of money so we can create new, more conscious relationships with money and with each other around money.

We follow certain core principles in the pursuit of change:

- Personal and social transformation are intimately connected.
- Personal transformation is greatly supported within small communities.
- The whole person — body, mind, emotion, and spirit — is engaged in a variety of methods for listening and knowing.
- Ideas are enriched and become useful through sharing and testing in action. We recognize that thinking is crucial, but we cannot just think our way into effective solutions to current global challenges.

All activities embodying these ideas occur with an awareness that there is a larger picture of reality, one that encompasses the unseen as well as the seen, one that honors the intelligence of the universe.

## Passion for exploring

The core of the Marion Foundation is a passion for exploring, for following a hunch that there is more to life than what fits into our everyday definition of reality. Programs and events include:

*Idea-sharing programs.* The foundation hosts gatherings from workshops to conferences on a variety of topics, periodically mailing selected articles and specially written pieces, offering books from a lending library, facilitating the publishing of selected books, and maintaining a website.

*Action-based programs.* We manage the affairs of the foundation using collaborative forms of decision-making that respect both reason and intuition. We engage with neighbors to create new possibilities in our local community, and we partner with individuals and groups who share the vision and leadership strength to affect systemic change in the larger world. In this last effort, we have developed a major program, Innovative Frontiers in Philanthropy, to connect individuals and groups with potential funders in new ways. Finally, we sponsor a Serendipity Fund to extend traditional funding boundaries by supporting individuals and ideas that stretch our imagination.

## Biological medicine

Biological medicine as practiced at the Paracelsus Klinik is one of the most truly holistic, integrative, and functional models of alternative medicine and healing in the world today. In 1999, the Marion Foundation joined with the Paracelsus Klinik in Switzerland and the Paracelsus Foxhollow Clinic in Kentucky to create the Biological Medicine Network (BMN).

Long available in Europe, biological medicine is now delivering benefits to countless North Americans, offering a comprehensive approach to medical care that enables individuals to take responsibility for their health and healing throughout life.

We invite you to learn more about the Marion Foundation. Our supplementary materials provide comprehensive descriptions of Marion Foundation activities.

Biological Medicine Network　　Phone: 508-748-0816
Marion Foundation, Inc.　　　　Fax: 508-748-1976
3 Barnabas Road　　　　　　　www.marionfoundation.org/
Marion, MA 02738　　　　　　　bookstore.asp
　　　　　　　　　　　　　　　bmn@marionfoundation.org

# Appendix B
## ABOUT THE PARACELSUS KLINIK   ·

THE PARACELSUS KLINIK in Lustmühle, Switzerland, was founded in 1958 as a center for health and well-being based on the principles of natural healing. Since then, it has integrated and adapted to evolving and developing models of biological and holistic medicine and dentistry.

The clinic's motivated team of about seventy-five health practitioners includes eight physicians, five dentists, several therapists, pharmacists, consultants from different scientific specializations, medical and dental assistants, dental technicians, and administrative assistants. Thus, a combination of treatments can be offered to meet the differing needs of patients.

The Paracelsus Klinik is the only outpatient clinic in Switzerland in which the full range of biological medicine is combined with conventional and state-of-the-art therapies designed to help balance and restore the overall regulation of the body's systems. This unique model also includes the integration of holistic dentistry.

In nearly all cases of acute and chronic disease, the patient can be either treated or advised on an outpatient or inpatient basis.

## Importance of dentistry

As it has been found through extensive study that the teeth as well as the jaw are frequently the cause for disease located elsewhere in the body, dental treatment is a key factor in this biological medicine system.

## On-site pharmacy

The on-site pharmacy at Paracelsus carries a complete range of biological supplements and medicines. The clinic also serves as an educational resource foundation for holistic medicine, offering further education to doctors, dentists, nonmedical practitioners, pharmacists, and other therapists.

## Beneficial treatment of acute and chronic disease

In addition to attending the clinic for preventive and health-maintenance reasons, people from all over the world choose Paracelsus because of its reputation for treating many different diseases very often without surgery. Many patients with breast and prostate cancer travel to the Paracelsus Klinik with beneficial results.

Chronic conditions like arthritis, asthma, allergies, endometriosis, and autoimmune diseases such as MS, Lyme disease and chronic fatigue are also commonly treated.

## Cost and other considerations

The optimal duration of a visit to the clinic can be anywhere from two to four weeks. Cost varies according to the amount and kind of dental work and supplements prescribed, as well as travel considerations and type of accommodations. The weekly cost of your visit may be between $3,000 to $5,000.(Higher costs occur when extensive dental work or additional therapies are required.) The length of stay varies from one week for preventive care to up to three weeks for chronic illnesses. Hotel information is included in our patient packet. Visit www.nfam.org and/or www.paracelsus.ch for more information.

# Glossary

**ALLOPATHIC** system of therapeutics in which diseases are treated by producing a condition that is incompatible with or antagonistic to the disease and its symptoms; conventional Western medicine is said to be allopathic.

**AYURVEDIC MEDICINE** theory that suggests that diseases of the body are caused by stresses in the awareness, or consciousness, of the individual; ayurvedic treatments include yoga-related body postures, breathing exercises, meditative techniques, special diets, and herbal remedies.

**BIOLOGICAL MEDICINE** holistic approach to health and wellness that allows the human body to maximize its own innate healing powers; combines traditional healing practices with modern, non-invasive diagnostic and treatment methods.

**BODYWORK** variety of techniques that promote relaxation and treat certain ailments, especially musculoskeletal disorders. Treatments include massage, movement awareness, structural realignment, and energy balancing.

**HOLISTIC** approach to medicine that assumes that the human being is a functioning system operating in a "state of wholeness"; holistic medicine views all aspects of an individual — physical, mental, emotional, and spiritual — as interrelated.

**HOMEOPATHY** therapeutic system in which diseases are treated by substances that can cause symptoms of disease in a healthy person but that, when administered in minute doses, can cure the same symptoms.

**KINESTHESIA**  the science of movement; in biological medicine, refers to movement and angles of joints that may be indicative of disease.

**NATUROPATHY**  system of medicine that treats health conditions by utilizing the body's inherent, natural ability to heal; diet, lifestyle, work, and personal history are all considered when determining a treatment regimen.

**NEURAL THERAPY**  injection of homeopathic remedies into the body's acupuncture points.

**OSTEOPATHY**  medical discipline that focuses on addressing problems in the musculoskeletal system to correct and improve the general functioning of the body.

**THERMOGRAPHY**  diagnostic technique that utilizes a thermalized (temperature-sensitive) wand, or thermister, to record skin temperature at 181 points on the body, first at standard room temperature, then at a lower temperature; responses provide feedback on functioning of organs and systems.

**TRADITIONAL CHINESE MEDICINE**  ancient system of holistic health care that uses a variety of treatments including acupressure, acupuncture, herbal therapies, and massage, along with health-sustaining energetic body movement such as tai chi.

# Resource List

## Videos

In this series of six videotapes, Dr. Thomas Rau explains biological medicine clearly and with passion and humor.

### *The Paradigms of Biological Medicine*

"To treat differently, you have to think differently," says Dr. Rau. Biological medicine is a comprehensive, holistic, integrative approach to health and illness. Rather than just looking at symptoms, biological medicine heals by finding the causes for disease in the body's regulatory systems.

### *Measuring Health: Regulation Test Methods*

To find internal dysfunctions, biological medicine uses different testing and diagnostic tools, some of which are not yet available in the United States. These devices, which measure the body's capacity to regulate its millions of functions, are able to help find the sources of disease.

### *Your Internal Environment, or Milieu*

Biological medicine looks at each individual on a cellular level. A healthy body wants to be in balance, but because of the influences of diet, toxins, bad air or water, stress, or even genetic weaknesses, our health and well-being can become unbalanced or diseased. By looking at the internal "milieu," biological medicine can diagnose these imbalances and begin to treat their causes.

### Cancer and Biological Medicine

The Paracelsus Klinik receives cancer patients from around the world. Dr. Rau describes cancer as a response to imbalances built up over years, many of which can be reversed with biological medicine. As with every disease, biological medicine looks for causes, unique in each patient, and develops treatment that corrects these internal malfunctions.

### Teeth and Illness

Dr. Rau explains the concepts of biological dentistry and the "dos and don'ts" of caring for your teeth, an essential part of treating illness in biological medicine. The Chinese meridian approach connects each tooth with various parts of the body. A tooth problem (infection, abscess, root canal, cavitation, amalgam fillings, and mercury) can cause illness somewhere else along its meridian.

### Allergies

Allergies have become a problem for more and more people. Dr. Rau explains why conventional medications only suppress symptoms temporarily, while a better understanding of food, diet, and exercise can cause them to disappear.

### To order videos, contact:

Marion Foundation, Inc.
3 Barnabas Road, Marion, MA 02738
Phone: (508) 748-0816
Fax: (508) 748-1976
www.marionfoundation.org/bookstore.asp

# Books

### Between Heaven and Earth: A Guide to Chinese Medicine
Harriet Beinfield and Efrem Korngold
Paperback
ISBN: 0345379748
Random House
1992

### The Complete Book of Chinese Health & Healing
Daniel Reid and Dexter Chow
Paperback
ISBN: 1570620717
Shambhala
1995

### Conscious Eating
Gabriel Cousens, MD
Paperback
ISBN: 1556432852
North Atlantic Books
2000

### Everybody's Guide to Homeopathic Medicines
Stephen Cummings, MD, and Dana Ullman, MPH
Paperback
ISBN: 0874778433
Putnam Publishing Group
1997

*Healing with Whole Foods: Oriental Traditions and
   Modern Nutrition*
Paul Pitchford
Paperback
ISBN: 1556432208
North Atlantic Books
1996


*Homeopathy: Medicine of the New Man*
George Vithoulkas
Paperback
Simon & Schuster
ISBN: 0671763288
1985


*Radical Healing: Integrating the World's Great Therapeutic
   Traditions to Create a New Transformative Medicine*
Rudolph M. Ballantine
Paperback
ISBN: 0609804847
Crown
2000


*Reclaiming the Wisdom of the Body: A Personal Guide to
   Chinese Medicine*
Sandra Hill
Paperback
ISBN: 0806520736
Carol
1999

*Root Canal Cover-Up*
George E. Meinig
Charlene Koonce and Mark Lovendale (Editors)
Paperback
ISBN: 0945196199
Bion
1994


*Theory and Practice of Biological Medicine*
David A. Edwards, MD, HMD
Paperback
ISBN: 0964732505
MG Reprographics
1995


*Tooth Truth*
Frank J. Jerome, DDS
Paperback
ISBN: 1890035130
New Century Press
2001


*The Toxic Time Bomb: Can the Mercury in Your Dental Fillings Poison You?*
Sam Ziff
Foreword by Jeffery Bland
Paperback
ISBN: 0943358248
Aurora Press
1985

*Uninformed Consent: The Hidden Dangers in Dental Care*
Hal A. Huggins and Thomas E. Levy
Paperback
ISBN: 1571741178
Hampton Roads
1998


*Whole Body Dentistry: Discover the Missing Piece to
    Better Health*
Mark A. Breiner with Foreword by Denise Dolence
Introduction by Robert C. Atkins
Paperback
ISBN: 0967844304
Quantum Health Press
1999